COMPLETE GUIDE TO GALLSTONES

A Comprehensive Handbook For Understanding, Preventing, Treating Cholelithiasis Naturally, Medically, Dietary Strategies, Symptoms Decoded And Surgery Insights

DEHART HAIRSTON

DISCLAIMER

This book's content is only intended for general informative purposes. At the time of writing, the author has taken every precaution to guarantee that the material is correct and current. Nevertheless, the author disclaims all explicit and implicit representations and guarantees about the availability, appropriateness, correctness, completeness, and usefulness of the material on these pages.

Since the author is not a licensed medical practitioner, the material in this book shouldn't be interpreted as medical advice. Before making any modifications to their diet, exercise regimen, or medical treatment, readers are urged to speak with a licensed healthcare provider.

Moreover, the author has no connection to any of the businesses, organizations, or people that are discussed in this book. Any mentions of goods, services, businesses, or people are purely informative and do not indicate endorsement or suggestion.

This book's content is entirely dependent on the author's expertise, study, and comprehension of the topic. Despite having taken reasonable care to offer correct information, the author disclaims all liability for any mistakes or omissions in the material as well as for any losses, harm, or damages resulting from using the information.

It is recommended that readers use their own judgment and discretion when applying the knowledge in this book to their own situations. The use or implementation of any material in this book may result in unfavorable repercussions, directly or indirectly, for which the author assumes no liability.

By reading this book, you agree to release and hold the author harmless from any claims, losses, liabilities, costs, or expenditures resulting from or related to the use of the information you get from it.

ABOUT THIS BOOK

"Gallstones: A Comprehensive Guide to Understanding, Preventing, and Managing" is an essential resource for anyone dealing with the complexities of gallstone-related health issues. With a meticulous breakdown of critical topics, this book ensures that readers have the knowledge they need to effectively address gallstone challenges.

Chapter 1 introduces readers to the fundamentals of gallstones, including their types, causes, and risk factors. Understanding these fundamentals lays the groundwork for understanding the following chapters, making it easier to grasp the complexities of gallstone management.

Chapter 2 delves into the anatomy of the gallbladder and biliary system, providing invaluable information about their functions and importance in digestion. With this knowledge, readers gain a better understanding of how gallstones affect bodily processes.

Moving on, Chapter 3 discusses the symptoms and diagnostic procedures associated with gallstones, empowering readers to recognize warning signs and seek prompt medical attention. Meanwhile, Chapter 4 discusses potential complications, emphasizing the critical importance of early detection and treatment for effective risk mitigation.

Chapter 5 discusses proactive gallstone prevention strategies, focusing on the role of diet, lifestyle changes, and weight management in reducing susceptibility. Subsequent chapters cover treatment options, post-treatment care, and long-term management, giving readers a comprehensive toolkit for navigating every stage of their gallstone journey.

Furthermore, the book goes beyond treatment and offers advice on how to live with gallstones, such as coping strategies, support resources, and prevention measures. This book serves as a beacon of hope and empowerment for those affected by gallstones, instilling confidence in readers to actively participate in their health journey.

Furthermore, Chapter 10 provides a glimpse into the future of gallstone treatment by highlighting current research and promising therapies. By staying informed and proactive, readers can look forward to a brighter, healthier future free of gallstone complications.

In essence, "Gallstones" is more than just a book; it's a lifeline for those dealing with gallstone-related issues, providing advice, support, and a road map to optimal health and well-being. With its comprehensive approach and invaluable insights, this book is a must-have for anyone looking to confidently navigate the complexities of gallstone management.

CHAPTER 1

Introduction To Gallstones

What Are Gallstones?

Gallstones are small, pebble-like structures that form in the gallbladder, a small organ beneath the liver. These stones are usually composed of cholesterol or bilirubin, a waste product produced by the liver. Gallstones can be as small as a grain of sand or as large as a golf ball, and they can number anywhere from one to several hundred.

Types Of Gallstones

There are two types of gallstones: cholesterol and pigment gallstones.

1. Cholesterol gallstones: These are the most common type of gallstones, accounting for roughly 80% of cases. They form when there is an imbalance in the components of bile, a digestive

fluid produced by the liver and stored in the gallbladder. When bile contains too much cholesterol and insufficient bile salts or lecithin to dissolve it, cholesterol crystallizes and forms stones.

2. Pigment gallstones: These stones are less common and are typically composed of bilirubin, a substance produced when red blood cells break down. Pigment gallstones are generally smaller and darker in color than cholesterol gallstones.

Causes And Risk Factors

Gallstones can form due to a variety of factors, including:

• Excess cholesterol in bile can crystallize and cause stones.

• Excess bilirubin can cause pigment gallstones.

• Impaired gallbladder function: Improper emptying or contraction can lead to bile concentration and stone formation.

• Obesity raises the risk of gallstones due to elevated cholesterol levels in bile.

• Rapid weight loss, such as crash dieting or bariatric surgery, may increase the risk of gallstones.

• Hormonal changes during pregnancy may increase the risk of gallstone formation.

• Certain medications, including birth control pills and cholesterol-lowering drugs, may increase the risk of gallstones.

• Gallstones are more likely to form in families, indicating a genetic predisposition.

Understanding these causes and risk factors is critical for identifying people who are more likely to develop gallstones and taking preventive measures to reduce their chances.

CHAPTER 2

Anatomy Of The Gallbladder And Biliary System

Understanding The Role Of The Gallbladder

The gallbladder is a small pear-shaped organ located beneath the liver on the upper right side of the abdomen. While it may appear insignificant, its function in digestion is critical. Consider it the body's storage facility for bile, the digestive fluid produced by the liver. When you eat a meal, particularly one high in fat, the gallbladder activates, releasing bile into the small intestine via a network of ducts.

This bile is required to break down fats into smaller molecules that can be absorbed and utilized by the body. Without enough bile, digestion becomes inefficient, resulting in discomfort and even serious health issues.

The gallbladder functions as a reservoir, storing bile between meals and releasing it when needed to aid digestion. Its capacity to control the flow of bile keeps the digestive process running smoothly, enabling nutrients to be absorbed properly.

Anatomy Of The Biliary System

To understand how the gallbladder fits into the bigger picture, you must first understand the biliary system's anatomy. This system includes the liver, gallbladder, and a network of ducts that carry bile from the liver to the small intestine. Imagine the liver as a powerhouse, constantly producing bile to aid digestion. Bile then passes via a variety of ducts, including the common hepatic and cystic ducts, before arriving at the gallbladder.

The gallbladder stores bile until it is required for digestion. When food reaches the small intestine, hormonal cues cause the gallbladder to contract and release bile into the digestive system. This concerted effort ensures that bile is given at the appropriate timing and volume to aid in fat breakdown.

Understanding the complex structure of the biliary system is critical for understanding how gallstones may impair normal function. When these small, hard deposits grow within the gallbladder, they may obstruct the flow of bile, causing discomfort, inflammation, and other issues.

Function Of Bile In Digestion

Bile has a varied function in digestion, acting as the body's natural detergent for breaking down fat. Bile, which is made up of water, bile salts, cholesterol, and waste materials, emulsifies fat globules, breaking them down into tiny droplets that enzymes can digest more easily.

Furthermore, bile assists in the absorption of fat-soluble vitamins including A, D, E, and K by enveloping them and transporting them across the intestinal wall. Without bile, these vital nutrients would pass through the digestive system unused, resulting in shortages and possible health consequences.

Beyond its function in fat digestion, bile aids in the elimination of waste products from the body, such as excess cholesterol and bilirubin, a result of red blood cell breakdown. Bile helps the body detoxify itself by delivering these toxins to the gut for elimination.

Bile is an important component of the digestive process, enabling fat breakdown and absorption while also assisting in waste disposal.

CHAPTER 3

Symptoms And Diagnosis

Common Symptoms Of Gallstones

Gallstones often lurk quietly, with no symptoms at all. When they do make their presence known, they might do so by several unsettling signals. One of the most prevalent symptoms is discomfort in the upper abdomen, usually on the right side. This discomfort may be intense and unexpected, especially after a meal, and it may spread to the back or shoulder blades. Others describe it as a clutching or cramping feeling.

Another distinguishing feature is jaundice, which appears as yellowing of the skin and eyes. This happens when gallstones block the bile duct, preventing bile from draining correctly into the intestines. Jaundice may also induce dark urine and pale feces as a result of bile flow disruptions.

Gallstones often cause nausea and vomiting, particularly when the pain is intense. Fatty or oily meals might increase these symptoms by causing the gallbladder to constrict, thereby worsening the obstruction caused by the stones.

In addition to these major symptoms, people with gallstones may have bloating, indigestion, and a sensitivity to fatty meals. Some people may feel full or uncomfortable in their belly, especially after eating a heavy meal.

It's crucial to remember that not everyone with gallstones will have symptoms, and the severity and frequency of symptoms might vary greatly from person to person. As a result, it's critical to monitor any changes in your body and get medical assistance if you have persistent or severe symptoms.

Diagnostic Procedures (Ultrasound, CT Scan, Blood Tests)

Gallstones are normally diagnosed using a combination of medical history, physical examination, and imaging testing. One of the most popular imaging procedures utilized is ultrasonography, which employs sound waves to generate pictures of the gallbladder and surrounding organs. Ultrasound is non-invasive, painless, and easily accessible, making it a great first-line diagnostic technique for gallstones.

In rare circumstances, a CT scan may be required to obtain more comprehensive views of the gallbladder and biliary system. CT scans employ a sequence of X-rays to produce cross-sectional pictures of the body, enabling healthcare practitioners to assess the size, location, and quantity of gallstones more precisely.

Blood tests may also be conducted to examine liver function and check for symptoms of inflammation or infection. Elevated levels of certain liver enzymes, such as alkaline phosphatase and bilirubin, may suggest bile duct blockage caused by gallstones.

Occasionally, further imaging tests such as magnetic resonance cholangiopancreatography (MRCP) or endoscopic retrograde cholangiopancreatography (ERCP) may be advised to further analyze the biliary system and prepare for future therapy.

When To Seek Medical Help

If you encounter symptoms indicative of gallstones, such as severe stomach pain, jaundice, or persistent nausea and vomiting, it's crucial to get medical care soon. While some instances of gallstones may be cured on their own without intervention, others may lead to problems such as inflammation of the gallbladder (cholecystitis), infection, or obstruction of the bile ducts.

Additionally, if you have a known history of gallstones and have a sudden onset of severe stomach discomfort, fever, or indications of infection, get emergency medical assistance since these might be indicators of a major complication needing urgent treatment.

Ignoring signs of gallstones may lead to greater discomfort and consequences, so it's always preferable to err on the side of caution and check with a healthcare expert if you have any concerns. Early identification and treatment may help avoid future problems and improve outcomes for persons with gallstones.

CHAPTER 4

Complications Of Gallstones

Gallstones, albeit little, may lead to major consequences if left untreated. Understanding these problems is vital for addressing gallstone-related diseases successfully.

Complications Such As Cholecystitis, Pancreatitis, And Jaundice

Cholecystitis occurs when gallstones clog the bile ducts, producing inflammation in the gallbladder. This inflammation may lead to severe stomach discomfort, nausea, vomiting, and fever. If left untreated, cholecystitis may proceed to more severe problems, such as infection or even gangrene of the gallbladder, which may demand emergency surgery to remove the affected organ.

Pancreatitis: Inflammation of the Pancreas

Gallstones may also induce pancreatitis by clogging the pancreatic duct, which delivers digesting enzymes from the pancreas to the small intestine. When this duct is clogged, digestive enzymes get trapped and begin to assault the pancreas itself, leading to inflammation and discomfort. Pancreatitis may vary from minor to life-threatening, with symptoms including severe stomach pain, nausea, vomiting, and fever. Prompt medical intervention is vital to avoid consequences such as infection, organ failure, or even death.

Jaundice: Yellowing of the Skin and Eyes

Jaundice is a typical consequence of gallstones that develop when bile passage from the liver to the small intestine is impeded by gallstones. When bile cannot adequately drain, it builds up in the circulation, resulting in yellowing of the skin and eyes, black urine, and pale feces.

Jaundice may be an indication of significant liver or gallbladder disorders and needs quick medical assessment to discover the underlying cause and proper treatment.

Long-Term Effects Of Untreated Gallstones

Ignoring gallstone symptoms or postponing treatment may have major long-term repercussions for your health. Chronic inflammation of the gallbladder or pancreas may lead to irreversible damage to these organs, increasing the risk of consequences such as recurrent infections, scarring, and reduced function. Untreated gallstones may also raise the chance of developing gallbladder or bile duct cancer over time. Additionally, continued gallstone-related symptoms may greatly influence your quality of life, leading to chronic discomfort, digestive difficulties, and nutritional deficiencies.

Importance Of Early Detection And Treatment

Early identification and treatment of gallstones are vital for avoiding problems and protecting your health. If you have symptoms such as severe abdomen pain, nausea, vomiting, or jaundice, get medical assistance soon. Your doctor may undertake testing, such as ultrasound or blood tests, to identify gallstones and establish the best course of therapy. In many situations, gallstones may be controlled with dietary adjustments, medication, or less invasive treatments such as laparoscopic surgery to remove the gallbladder. Early management may help avoid problems, improve symptoms, and lessen the chance of long-term harm to your health. Don't overlook the warning signals of gallstones—talk to your doctor and take action to preserve your well-being.

CHAPTER 5

Prevention Strategies

Dietary Recommendations To Prevent Gallstones

Diet has a significant part in avoiding gallstones. By making sensible decisions, you may dramatically lower your chance of acquiring them. One of the primary nutritional suggestions is to have a balanced diet that includes lots of fruits, vegetables, healthy grains, and lean meats. These foods are rich in fiber, vitamins, and minerals, which support overall digestive health and may help reduce the production of gallstones.

In addition to including nutritious foods in your diet, it's crucial to restrict the intake of certain kinds of fats, notably saturated and trans fats. These fats are present in many processed and fried meals, as well as fatty cuts of meat and full-fat dairy products. Instead, go for healthy fats such as those found in olive oil, avocados, and nuts, which may help lower cholesterol levels and lessen the chance of gallstone development.

Another dietary tip for avoiding gallstones is to restrict your consumption of cholesterol-rich foods. High amounts of cholesterol in the bile may lead to the production of gallstones. To keep your cholesterol levels in control, restrict your intake of foods like red meat, eggs, and high-fat dairy items. Instead, concentrate on including more plant-based foods in your diet, such as beans, lentils, and healthy grains.

Lastly, keeping hydrated is vital for avoiding gallstones. Drinking enough of water throughout the day helps maintain bile moving smoothly through the gallbladder and decreases the danger of bile being excessively concentrated, which may contribute to the creation of gallstones.

Aim to drink at least eight glasses of water a day, and consider adding lemon or lime to your water for an added dose of digestive health.

Lifestyle Changes To Reduce The Risk

In addition to food alterations, some lifestyle changes may also help minimize the chance of getting gallstones. One of the most crucial lifestyle modifications is to maintain a healthy weight. Being overweight or obese raises the chance of gallstones, therefore lowering weight if you're carrying additional pounds may drastically lessen your risk.

Regular physical exercise is another key component of gallstone prevention. Exercise not only helps with weight control but also improves general digestive health and decreases cholesterol levels in the blood. Aim for at least 30 minutes of moderate-intensity activity most days of the week, such as brisk walking, cycling, or swimming.

Managing stress is also crucial for avoiding gallstones. Chronic stress may disturb the digestive process and lead to abnormalities in bile production and flow, increasing the risk of gallstone development. Incorporating stress-reducing activities into your daily routine, such as meditation, yoga, or deep breathing exercises, may help maintain your digestive system running smoothly and minimize your risk of gallstones.

Lastly, avoid crash diets or quick weight reduction programs, since they might increase the chance of gallstone development. Instead, concentrate on making incremental, lasting adjustments to your diet and lifestyle that support long-term health and well-being.

Importance Of Maintaining A Healthy Weight

Maintaining a healthy weight is vital for avoiding gallstones and supporting overall health. Excess weight, especially around the waistline, raises the risk of gallstone development by forcing the liver to create more cholesterol, which may contribute to the creation of gallstones.

Losing weight if you're overweight or obese may dramatically lessen your chances of acquiring gallstones. Even small weight reduction might have a substantial influence on gallstone prevention. Aim to lose weight gradually, at a pace of around 1-2 pounds per week, using a mix of good food and frequent activity.

In addition to avoiding gallstones, keeping a healthy weight decreases the risk of several other chronic conditions, including heart disease, diabetes, and some forms of cancer.

By adopting a healthy lifestyle that includes a balanced diet, regular exercise, and stress management skills, you may not only avoid gallstones but also enhance your general health and well-being for years to come.

CHAPTER 6

Treatment Options

Non-Surgical Approaches (Medications, Dissolution Therapy)

Non-surgical treatment options for gallstones provide a less intrusive method for people who may not be acceptable candidates for surgery or wish to explore alternatives first. Medications might be provided to help dissolve gallstones over time. These drugs often include bile acids, which act by gradually breaking down the cholesterol in the gallstones, enabling them to be discharged naturally via the bile ducts.

One typical medicine used for dissolving treatment is ursodeoxycholic acid (UDCA). UDCA helps to lower the cholesterol content of gallstones and may prevent new ones from developing.

However, it's crucial to realize that dissolution treatment may be a long process, frequently requiring months or even years to see substantial improvements. Additionally, not all kinds of gallstones react well to this therapy, especially those formed predominantly of calcium or pigment.

Patients receiving dissolution therapy will need frequent monitoring using imaging tests, such as ultrasound, to follow the course of the treatment and ensure the gallstones are decreasing adequately. While non-surgical treatments like dissolution therapy may be intriguing to some owing to their less intrusive nature, it's vital to examine the possible risks and benefits with your healthcare physician to see whether this choice is acceptable for your unique situation.

Surgical Options (Cholecystectomy)

Surgery, primarily cholecystectomy, is the most frequent and effective therapy for gallstones, particularly for individuals having symptoms or problems. Cholecystectomy entails the surgical removal of the gallbladder, where the gallstones are normally situated. There are two basic procedures for conducting cholecystectomy: laparoscopic and open surgery.

Laparoscopic cholecystectomy is the recommended option in most situations owing to its less invasive nature and quicker recovery time compared to open surgery. During a laparoscopic operation, small incisions are created in the belly, and a tiny camera (laparoscope) and surgical equipment are introduced to remove the gallbladder.

Open cholecystectomy, on the other hand, entails a bigger incision in the belly to reach and remove the gallbladder directly. While this procedure may be essential in some cases, such as if there are issues or difficulties with laparoscopic surgery, it often involves a longer recovery time and may result in greater pain and scars.

Before having cholecystectomy, patients will have pre-operative evaluations to evaluate their general health and any possible hazards related to the procedure. Your healthcare professional will describe the process in detail, including what to anticipate before, during, and after surgery, as well as any possible issues or side effects.

Risks And Benefits Of Each Treatment Option

When contemplating treatment options for gallstones, it's vital to examine the risks and advantages of each therapy carefully. Non-surgical alternatives including pharmaceutical therapy may be helpful for certain individuals, giving a less intrusive alternative to surgery. However, these therapies may take time to be successful and may not be suited for all kinds of gallstones.

Surgical procedures, notably cholecystectomy, are often extremely efficient in relieving symptoms and preventing future problems associated with gallstones. However, surgery brings its own set of dangers, including those connected with anesthesia, infection, bleeding, and harm to neighboring organs. Additionally, some individuals may develop digestive problems or bile reflux following gallbladder removal.

Your healthcare professional will work with you to analyze your unique condition, taking into consideration aspects such as the size and composition of your gallstones, your general health, and your personal preferences.

Together, you can make an educated choice on the best treatment option for treating your gallstones and increasing your quality of life. Regular follow-up sessions will be planned to evaluate your progress and handle any concerns or difficulties that may develop.

CHAPTER 7

Recovery And Post-Treatment Care

What To Expect After Gallbladder Surgery

Gallbladder surgery, also known as cholecystectomy, is a frequent treatment done to remove the gallbladder, generally owing to the presence of gallstones. After the operation, it's typical to endure some pain and changes while your body adjusts to the removal of the gallbladder. Here's what you may anticipate throughout the rehabilitation process:

1. **Hospital remains:** Depending on the kind of surgery (laparoscopic or open) and your general health, you may remain in the hospital for a day or two after the operation. During this period, medical professionals will check your status and give pain treatment as required.

2. Pain & Discomfort: It's usual to suffer some pain and discomfort in the abdomen, shoulder, or back after surgery. Your healthcare staff will prescribe pain medication to assist control any discomfort. Over time, the discomfort should progressively reduce as you recuperate.

3. Activity Level: While it's vital to relax and allow your body to recuperate, it's equally crucial to gradually raise your activity level. Your healthcare physician will offer advice on when it's safe to resume typical activities, including work, exercise, and driving.

4. Dietary Changes: After gallbladder surgery, you may need to make modifications to your diet to accommodate the loss of the gallbladder. This may involve gradually reintroducing solid meals, avoiding fatty or oily foods that might cause digestive pain, and increasing your consumption of fiber-rich foods to promote digestion.

 You will likely have a follow-up consultation with your surgeon to check your progress and discuss any concerns or issues you may have. It's vital to attend these visits and follow any suggestions supplied by your healthcare team.

Overall, although recovery following gallbladder surgery may take some time, most patients can resume their typical activities within a few weeks. By following your healthcare provider's advice and taking care of yourself, you may support a smooth recovery process.

Dietary Modifications Post-Treatment

Following gallbladder surgery, adopting dietary alterations might assist promote your recovery and prevent digestive pain. Here are some ideas for modifying your diet post-treatment:

1. Gradual Introduction of items: After surgery, start with a bland diet consisting of readily digested items such as broth, applesauce, and crackers. Gradually reintroduce solid meals, starting with low-fat alternatives such as lean meats, fruits, vegetables, and whole grains.

2. Limit Fatty meals: Since the gallbladder is crucial for storing and releasing bile to help in the digestion of fats, you may encounter trouble digesting fatty or greasy meals following surgery. Limit your consumption of high-fat meals such as fried dishes, creamy sauces, and fatty cuts of meat.

3. Increase Fiber Intake: Fiber-rich meals may help support good digestion and reduce constipation, which is common following gallbladder surgery. Include lots of fruits, vegetables, legumes, and whole grains in your diet to guarantee a sufficient fiber intake.

4. Stay Hydrated: Drinking enough of water is vital for avoiding dehydration and improving digestion.

Aim to drink at least eight glasses of water each day and restrict your consumption of caffeinated and alcoholic drinks, which may irritate the digestive system.

5. Monitor Symptoms: Pay attention to how your body responds to particular meals and make modifications appropriately. If you feel digestive pain, bloating, or diarrhea after eating particular foods, try removing them from your diet or ingesting them in smaller doses.

By adopting moderate dietary alterations and following your body's signals, you may assist promote your recovery and reduce digestive difficulties after gallbladder surgery.

Tips For Managing Discomfort And Promoting Healing

While discomfort is typical following gallbladder surgery, there are numerous tactics you may employ to control pain and promote healing throughout the recovery period. Here are some ways to help you feel more comfortable:

1. Take Pain Medication as Prescribed: Your healthcare practitioner will prescribe pain medication to assist manage post-surgery discomfort. Take your medicine as advised, and don't hesitate to contact your healthcare provider if you feel severe or chronic discomfort.

2. Apply Heat: Applying a heating pad or warm compress to the belly will help decrease muscular pain and discomfort. Just be careful to select a low or medium heat setting and avoid putting the heating pad directly on your skin to prevent burns.

3. Practice Deep Breathing: Deep breathing techniques may help decrease stress, relax stiff muscles, and improve healing.

Take slow, deep breaths, concentrating on extending your diaphragm and filling your lungs with air.

4. Get Plenty of Rest: Adequate rest is vital for helping your body to recuperate properly following surgery. Aim to get enough of sleep and take short naps during the day as required. Avoid intense activity that might strain your abdominal muscles.

5. Stay Positive: Maintaining a positive attitude may assist minimize stress and enhance a feeling of well-being throughout the healing process. Surround yourself with supportive friends and family members, and don't hesitate to ask for assistance when you need it.

By following these recommendations and listening to your body's demands, you may successfully manage pain and promote healing throughout your recovery after gallbladder surgery.

CHAPTER 8

Living With Gallstones

Coping Strategies For Living With Gallstones

Living with gallstones may be tough, but with the correct coping skills, it's possible to manage symptoms and retain a high quality of life. One of the most crucial coping methods is recognizing your illness. Educate yourself about gallstones, including their causes, symptoms, and treatment options. This information will allow you to make educated choices about your health and seek appropriate treatment when required.

Another key coping approach is adopting nutritional modifications. Certain foods may induce gallstone symptoms, therefore it's vital to avoid these meals and concentrate on a diet that is low in fat and cholesterol. This may involve including more fruits, vegetables, and healthy grains in your meals while decreasing your consumption of greasy and fried foods.

Staying hydrated is also vital for controlling gallstones. Drinking lots of water may help prevent the growth of gallstones and ease symptoms like pain and discomfort. Aim to drink at least eight glasses of water a day, and consider taking a water bottle with you to remain hydrated throughout the day.

Managing stress is another crucial coping tactic for living with gallstones. Stress may increase symptoms and make them harder to live with. Practice relaxation methods such as deep breathing, meditation, or yoga to help decrease tension and generate a feeling of peace.

It's also crucial to listen to your body and pace yourself correctly. Know your boundaries and avoid overexerting yourself, particularly during flare-ups of symptoms. Be careful to obtain a proper amount of rest and emphasize self-care activities that enhance general well-being.

Lastly, don't hesitate to seek help from friends, family, or a support group. Living with a chronic ailment like gallstones may seem isolated at times, but connecting with people who are going through similar circumstances can bring comfort and support. Reach out to loved ones for emotional support, and consider joining a support group where you can share your problems and achievements with people who understand.

Long-Term Management And Monitoring

Managing gallstones is not only about treating symptoms; it's also about long-term maintenance and monitoring to avoid problems and preserve general health.

After obtaining treatment for gallstones, whether by medication, lifestyle modifications, or surgery, it's crucial to follow up with your healthcare practitioner periodically for monitoring and assessment.

Long-term care may entail frequent check-ups, imaging tests, and blood work to monitor the health of your gallbladder and identify any possible concerns early on. Your healthcare professional may also prescribe continuous dietary and lifestyle adjustments to prevent the production of new gallstones and lower the chance of recurrence.

In rare circumstances, long-term therapy may also involve medicine to assist dissolve gallstones or prevent their development. These drugs act by lowering the quantity of cholesterol or bile acids in the bile, hence decreasing the risk of gallstone development. Your healthcare professional will pick the most suitable drug based on your unique requirements and medical history.

It's crucial to be proactive and cautious about your health while treating gallstones long-term. Pay attention to any changes in symptoms or new symptoms that may occur, and don't hesitate to contact your healthcare professional if you have any concerns. By keeping proactive and working closely with your healthcare team, you may successfully treat gallstones and limit the risk of complications.

Support Resources For Patients And Caregivers

Living with gallstones might be difficult, but you don't have to tackle it alone. There are several support options available for both patients and caregivers to offer advice, knowledge, and emotional support along the process.

One important resource is patient advocacy groups focused on gallbladder health. These organizations generally include instructional materials, online forums, and support groups where patients and caregivers may interact with others experiencing similar issues. They may also give tools for identifying healthcare experts specialized in gallbladder diseases and information about the latest research and treatment choices.

Online networks and social media groups may also be valuable sources of support for patients and caregivers. These virtual communities give a forum for sharing experiences, asking questions, and delivering encouragement in a secure and friendly atmosphere. Connecting with individuals who understand what you're going through may help ease feelings of loneliness and give vital insights and guidance.

Additionally, healthcare practitioners and medical institutes may provide support services for patients and caregivers living with gallstones. These services may include psychotherapy, dietary counseling, and access to further resources and referrals as required. Don't hesitate to call out your healthcare physician or medical institution to learn about available support services.

Finally, don't underestimate the importance of support from friends and family. Having a solid support network may make a major difference in your capacity to manage gallstones and handle the problems that come with maintaining a chronic disease. Don't be hesitant to count on your loved ones for emotional support, practical help, and encouragement along the process.

CHAPTER 9

Complications And Recurrence Prevention

Strategies To Prevent Recurrence Of Gallstones

Preventing the recurrence of gallstones is crucial to preserving long-term health and preventing future difficulties. While treatment options like surgery or medication may remove current gallstones, it's vital to implement lifestyle modifications to avoid their reappearance.

Dietary adjustments have a crucial influence in reducing gallstone recurrence. A diet rich in fiber, fruits, vegetables, and whole grains may help manage cholesterol levels in the bile, minimizing the probability of gallstone development. Avoiding high-fat, high-cholesterol diets may also minimize the incidence of gallstone recurrence.

Hydration is another crucial aspect of avoiding gallstones. Drinking a proper quantity of water every day helps keep bile diluted and reduces the development of cholesterol and other chemicals that lead to gallstone formation. Aim to drink at least eight glasses of water a day to maintain healthy hydration levels.

Maintaining a healthy weight is vital for avoiding gallstone recurrence. Obesity is a substantial risk factor for gallstone development, thus participating in regular physical exercise and adopting a balanced diet will help control weight and lower the chance of recurrence.

Monitoring For Complications Post-Treatment

After getting treatment for gallstones, it's crucial to monitor for any possible consequences to guarantee quick intervention and avoid any health difficulties. While most treatment approaches are typically safe, problems may nonetheless emerge in certain circumstances.

One typical consequence after gallstone therapy is infection. Infections may arise at the site of operation or in the bile ducts, leading to symptoms such as fever, stomach discomfort, and jaundice. Prompt detection and treatment of infections are critical to avoid future problems.

Another possible risk is bile duct damage or leaking. This may occur during surgical treatments to remove gallstones or during the implantation of stents to unblock clogged bile ducts. Symptoms of bile duct damage include severe stomach discomfort, fever, and jaundice. Immediate medical assistance is essential if these symptoms arise.

Monitoring for problems also entails frequent follow-up visits with healthcare specialists. During these visits, healthcare providers may examine the patient's healing status, address any concerns or symptoms, and request more testing if required. Following the prescribed follow-up program ensures that any issues are discovered early and addressed efficiently.

When To Follow Up With Healthcare Providers

Knowing when to follow up with healthcare experts is critical for ensuring good recovery and avoiding problems. The time and frequency of follow-up visits may vary based on the kind of therapy received and specific patient characteristics.

Generally, patients should plan a follow-up consultation with their healthcare physician within a few weeks after receiving gallstone therapy. During this first session, the healthcare professional may assess the patient's recovery progress, address any post-treatment symptoms or concerns, and discuss long-term management measures.

Subsequent follow-up appointments may be planned depending on the patient's condition and treatment plan. Patients with a history of gallstones or underlying health issues may need more regular monitoring to avoid recurrence and discover consequences early.

Individuals must speak honestly with their healthcare providers and report any new or worsening symptoms between follow-up appointments. Promptly seeking medical assistance for any worrying symptoms might help avoid problems and guarantee optimum results.

CHAPTER 10

Future Outlook And Advances In Treatment

Current Research And Advancements In Gallstone Treatment

In the domain of gallstone therapy, continuing research and developments are constantly redefining the landscape, bringing hope and answers to those suffering from this problem. Scientists and medical experts are devoted to understanding the complexity of gallstones, pursuing creative techniques for diagnosis, therapy, and finally, prevention.

One key area of interest in current research includes investigating the underlying causes and risk factors linked with gallstone development. By diving into the complicated processes that lead to the formation of gallstones, researchers seek to uncover new treatment targets and approaches.

This multimodal approach incorporates genetic predispositions, lifestyle variables, dietary habits, and the involvement of gut bacteria in gallstone etiology.

Advancements in diagnostic methods reflect another crucial component of modern gallstone research. Traditional approaches such as ultrasonic imaging remain crucial in identifying gallstones, although modern technologies provide greater precision and accuracy. From magnetic resonance imaging (MRI) to computed tomography (CT) scans, these modern imaging modalities provide doctors with a full perspective of gallstone-related disease, supporting better-informed treatment choices.

Furthermore, there is a concentrated effort to enhance current therapy procedures and create new approaches for gallstone breakdown and removal. While surgical treatments like laparoscopic cholecystectomy remain the gold standard for gallstone therapy, less invasive approaches continue to advance, lowering patient morbidity and boosting recovery times. Additionally, pharmaceutical treatments aiming at dissolving cholesterol-based gallstones are being extensively studied, presenting a non-surgical option for select patients.

In combination with these therapeutic improvements, there is a rising focus on individualized therapy in the domain of gallstone treatment. Tailoring therapy regimens to unique patient profiles, including genetic predispositions and comorbidities, offers tremendous potential for maximizing treatment results and avoiding unwanted effects. Through a full knowledge of the patient's specific physiological composition, doctors may personalize therapies to address the fundamental causes of gallstone development, promoting more effective and durable results.

As research in the area of gallstone therapy continues to improve, both healthcare professionals and patients alike must remain educated and proactive. By being aware of the newest breakthroughs and treatment approaches, people may make empowered choices on their healthcare journey. Moreover, continued involvement in clinical trials and research activities allows patients to contribute to the collective knowledge base, promoting innovation and improvement in gallstone therapy.

Promising Therapies On The Horizon

The horizon of gallstone therapy brims with promise, as researchers explore fresh therapeutic options and inventive methods to tackling this ubiquitous illness. From innovative pharmacological drugs to cutting-edge surgical approaches, several potential treatments are at the forefront of changing gallstone care, bringing newfound hope to patients tormented by this condition.

One of the most anticipated advancements in gallstone treatment includes the emergence of pharmacological medicines targeted to dissolve cholesterol-based gallstones. These drugs, known as oral bile acid treatments, act by modifying the composition of bile, so encouraging the breakdown of cholesterol crystals inside the gallbladder. By utilizing the body's natural systems for bile metabolism, these drugs provide a non-invasive option to surgical intervention, especially for those with symptomatic gallstones who are reluctant to surgery or judged unsuitable candidates.

Furthermore, the field of endoscopic retrograde cholangiopancreatography (ERCP) continues to undergo advancements, opening the door for less invasive techniques for gallstone removal. With the introduction of improved endoscopic procedures and instruments, doctors may now safely traverse the convoluted biliary path, aiding the extraction of gallstones stuck inside the common bile duct. This strategy not only obviates the need for open surgery but also mitigates the risk of postoperative problems, giving a safer and more efficient option for chosen individuals.

In addition to these treatment techniques, the developing area of lithotripsy shows tremendous potential for the non-invasive therapy of gallstones. Extracorporeal shock wave lithotripsy (ESWL), initially designed for the treatment of renal calculi, has received interest as a possible method for gallstone fragmentation. By administering concentrated shock waves to the gallbladder, ESWL compromises gallstone integrity, enabling their transit through the biliary system and subsequent elimination. This non-surgical technique provides a compelling option for those with symptomatic gallstones who prefer to avoid invasive treatments or are judged unsuitable candidates for surgery.

As these promising medicines inch closer to clinical adoption, healthcare practitioners and patients alike need to stay cautious and educated. By adopting these novel techniques and engaging in current research activities, people may actively contribute to the improvement of gallstone therapy, ushering in a new age of individualized, patient-centered care.

Encouragement For Staying Informed And Proactive

In the ever-evolving environment of gallstone therapy, remaining educated and proactive is important to obtaining maximum health outcomes and quality of life. As new research results emerge and breakthrough medicines come to fruition, people are encouraged to take an active part in managing their gallstone-related difficulties, equipped with information and awareness.

One of the most efficient methods to keep informed is by having open and proactive contact with healthcare professionals. By participating in meaningful discourse with doctors and experts, people may obtain vital insights into the newest breakthroughs in gallstone therapy, as well as individualized advice suited to their particular medical history and preferences. Moreover, looking out for credible sources of knowledge, such as medical publications, professional associations, and recognized websites, helps people to remain updated on current advances and developing medicines in the area.

Furthermore, establishing a proactive attitude to healthcare requires accepting lifestyle alterations and preventative treatments targeted at minimizing the risk of gallstone development and recurrence.

Adopting a balanced diet rich in fruits, vegetables, whole grains, and lean proteins, while minimizing saturated fats and processed carbohydrates, plays a significant role in maintaining good gallbladder health. Regular physical exercise, weight control, and reduction in alcohol intake also contribute to general well-being and may lower the probability of gallstone-related problems.

Additionally, those with a tendency to gallstone development, such as those with a family history of gallstones or certain medical conditions, may benefit from proactive screening and risk assessment. By working together with healthcare practitioners to identify possible risk factors and adopting preventative methods early on, people may decrease the chance of gallstone-related problems and improve long-term health outcomes.

In conclusion, by keeping educated, proactive, and involved in their healthcare journey, people may negotiate the intricacies of gallstone therapy with confidence and resilience. Through continued education, advocacy, and cooperation with healthcare practitioners, people may empower themselves to make educated choices and embrace novel medicines that give hope and healing in the face of gallstone-related issues.

CONCLUSION

In conclusion, gallstones constitute a frequent but potentially deadly medical problem impacting millions globally. Through this examination, it becomes obvious that knowing their genesis, symptoms, diagnostic procedures, and therapy alternatives is crucial in treating this illness properly.

Gallstones arise via a complicated interaction of variables such as heredity, nutrition, obesity, and cholesterol metabolism. Their existence may lead to a range of symptoms ranging from modest pain to serious consequences such as cholecystitis, pancreatitis, or even gallbladder cancer. Early identification by imaging modalities like ultrasonography, CT scans, or MRI is critical for quick action.

Treatment options for gallstones include lifestyle adjustments, medication, and surgical intervention.

While non-surgical alternatives like medication or lithotripsy may be acceptable for certain people, surgical removal of the gallbladder (cholecystectomy) remains the gold standard for those with symptomatic gallstones or problems. Laparoscopic cholecystectomy has become the preferred surgical method owing to its less invasive nature and faster recovery duration.

Moreover, preventative methods play a key role in decreasing the risk of gallstone development. These include maintaining a healthy weight, eating a balanced diet high in fiber and low in saturated fats, keeping hydrated, and avoiding quick weight reduction regimes. Regular physical exercise also aids in gallstone prevention by enhancing overall metabolic health.

Furthermore, continuing research continues to deepen our knowledge of gallstone pathogenesis and create innovative treatment methods.

Future developments may lead to more tailored therapies, possibly lowering the burden of gallstone-related illness and death.

Although gallstones represent substantial health difficulties, proactive treatment via a mix of lifestyle adjustments, early identification, and appropriate therapies may help improve outcomes and increase the quality of life for persons afflicted by this illness.

THE END